The ABCs of Why It's Not Good For Men to be Alone

(and This Includes Women)

Louis Dace

ISBN 979-8-89043-334-3 (paperback)
ISBN 979-8-89043-335-0 (digital)

Christian Faith Publishing
832 Park Avenue
Meadville, PA 16335
www.christianfaithpublishing.com

Printed in the United States of America

CONTENTS

FOREWORD

(A) Almighty God

In the beginning God created the heavens and earth! And, God said "Let there be light" and there was light! God saw that the light was good!

And, God said "Let the waters under the sky be gathered to one place and let the dry ground appear." And, God saw that it was good!

Then, God said "Let the land produce vegetation; seed-bearing plants and trees on the land that bear fruit with seed in it according to their various kind" and it was so. And God saw that it was good!

And, God said "Let there be lights in the expanse of the sky to separate the day from the night and let them serve as signs to mark seasons and days and years—God made two great lights.

The greater light to govern the day and the lesser light to govern the night. He also made the stars, God set them in the sky to give light on the earth, to govern the day and the night and to separate light from darkness. And, God saw that it was good!

And, God said let the waters team with living creatures and let the birds fly above the earth across the sky. So God created the great creatures of the sea and every living and moving thing in the waters and every winged bird according to their kind. And, God saw that it was good!

And, God said "Let the land produce living creatures according to their kind" And, God saw that it was good!

Then God said "Let us make Man in our image, in our likeness, and let him rule over the fish of the sea and the birds of the air, and over every living creature that moves on the ground.

Then, God said "It is NOT good for man to be alone, I will make for him a partner suitable for him!" For this reason a man will leave his father and mother and be united to his wife and they will become one!

(B) Blessings

> Blessed is the person that finds their mate. Enjoy life with your mate, whom you love, all the days of this meaningless life that God has given you under the sun—all your meaningless days. For this is your lot in life and in your toilsome labor under the sun. (Ecclesiastes 9:9)

(C) Community

Communications, children, and cycles.

CHAPTER 1

Introduction

The importance of relationships

Relationships are an essential part of human life and play a vital role in our physical, mental, and emotional well-being. Human beings are social animals, and as such, we have a natural need for social connections and relationships.

Having healthy relationships with family, friends, romantic partners, and even coworkers can provide a sense of belonging, support, and comfort. Our relationships can also impact our self-esteem, confidence, and sense of identity. In addition, having a network of relationships can provide opportunities for personal growth and development.

Research has shown that strong social connections and relationships can have significant health benefits, including reducing stress, improving cardiovascular health, and boosting our immune system. Additionally, individuals with strong social networks tend to live longer and experience a higher quality of life than those who are socially isolated.

In summary, the importance of relationships lies in their ability to provide support, comfort, and belonging as well as contribute to our overall well-being and health.

The impact of isolation on men and women

Isolation can have a profound impact on the mental, physical, and emotional well-being of both men and women. Here are some specific ways isolation can affect men and women:

1. *Mental health.* Isolation can lead to increased feelings of loneliness, anxiety, and depression in both men and women. This can be especially true for those who are socially isolated for long periods. The lack of social interaction can also exacerbate existing mental health conditions, such as bipolar disorder and schizophrenia.
2. *Physical health.* Isolation has been linked to an increased risk of chronic conditions such as heart disease, high blood pressure, and diabetes. Additionally, socially isolated individuals are more likely to engage in unhealthy behaviors, such as overeating, lack of physical exercise, and drug and alcohol abuse.
3. *Relationships.* Men and women who are isolated may have fewer opportunities to form meaningful relationships with others, whether it be romantic, platonic, or familial. This can lead to a lack of emotional support and increased feelings of loneliness.
4. *Career.* Isolation can impact career success. A lack of social interaction can limit opportunities for networking, collaboration, and learning from others in the workplace.
5. *Quality of life.* Isolation can lead to a decreased quality of life. Social interaction provides a sense of purpose and meaning, and the absence of this can lead to feelings of hopelessness and helplessness.

In summary, the impact of isolation on men and women can be significant and multifaceted, affecting mental and physical health, relationships, career, and overall quality of life. It's important for individuals to prioritize their social connections to maintain their well-being.

THE ABCS OF WHY IT'S NOT GOOD FOR MEN TO BE ALONE (AND THIS INCLUDES WOMEN)

The purpose of the book

The purpose of the book *The ABCs of Why It's Not Good for Men to Be Alone (And This Includes Women)* is to explore the various ways social isolation and loneliness can negatively impact the lives of both men and women. The book aims to provide insight into the psychological, physical, and social effects of isolation and highlight the importance of maintaining healthy relationships.

The book is designed to be a comprehensive guide for readers who are interested in learning more about the negative impacts of isolation and the benefits of healthy relationships. It aims to provide a clear understanding of the biology and psychology behind human connections and highlight the positive effects of social support.

Through exploring the history and science of human connection, the book aims to provide a convincing argument for the importance of social interaction and the detrimental effects of isolation. Additionally, the book will provide practical advice and guidance for readers who are looking to build and maintain healthy relationships in their own lives.

Overall, the purpose of this book is to provide a comprehensive exploration of the impact of isolation and the benefits of social interaction, with the ultimate goal of helping readers lead happier, healthier, and more fulfilling lives.

CHAPTER 2

The History of Human Connection

The evolution of social behavior

THE EVOLUTION OF social behavior is a complex topic, and many factors have contributed to the development of social behavior over time. In general, social behavior has evolved as a way for individuals to survive and reproduce more effectively. Here are some of the key factors that have contributed to the evolution of social behavior:

1. *Natural selection.* Social behavior has evolved through the process of natural selection. Over time, individuals who have developed successful social strategies that enable them to survive and reproduce more effectively are more likely to pass on their genes to future generations.

2. *Group living.* Living in groups can provide many benefits, such as protection from predators, access to food and resources, and the opportunity to mate. Social behavior has evolved as a way to help individuals live together in groups, cooperate with one another, and avoid conflict.

3. *Communication.* The development of communication, such as language and gestures, has played a critical role in the evolution of social behavior. Communication allows individuals to coordinate their actions, share information, and form alliances.

4. *Competition.* Competition for resources, mates, and other factors has also played a role in the evolution of social behavior. Social strategies that allow individuals to compete more effectively, such as forming alliances or cooperating with kin, have evolved over time.

5. *Cognition.* Finally, the evolution of social behavior has also been influenced by cognitive abilities, such as the ability to understand and anticipate the behavior of others. Individuals who are better able to understand and navigate complex social dynamics are more likely to survive and reproduce.

In summary, the evolution of social behavior has been influenced by a range of factors, including natural selection, group living, communication, competition, and cognition. Understanding the development of social behavior over time can help us better understand human behavior and the role of social interaction in our lives.

The role of communities in early human societies

The role of communities in early human societies was critical for survival, and it played a key role in shaping human behavior and culture. Here are some of the ways that communities were important in early human societies:

1. *Protection.* Living in a community provided safety and protection from predators and other dangers. Early humans lived in groups, and they worked together to protect themselves and their resources.

2. *Sharing resources.* Communities also facilitated the sharing of resources, such as food, water, and shelter. Early humans

shared resources to ensure that everyone in the group had access to what they needed to survive.

3. *Socialization.* Communities provided opportunities for socialization, learning, and the development of culture. Early humans lived in groups, and they shared knowledge and skills with one another. This facilitated the development of complex language, tools, and other cultural practices.

4. *Reproduction.* Communities were also critical for reproduction. Early humans lived in small groups, and they formed intimate social relationships with one another. This facilitated mate selection, child-rearing, and the passing on of cultural traditions to future generations.

5. *Identity.* Communities provided a sense of identity and belonging for early humans. Living in a community meant that individuals had a place within a larger social structure, which provided them with a sense of purpose and meaning.

In summary, communities played a critical role in early human societies. It facilitated safety and protection, the sharing of resources, socialization, reproduction, and identity. Understanding the role of communities in early human societies can help us better understand the evolution of human behavior and culture.

The impact of industrialization on social structures

The impact of industrialization on social structures was profound and far-reaching. As industrialization spread across the world in the eighteenth and nineteenth centuries, traditional social structures were upended, and new forms of social organization emerged. Here are some of the ways that industrialization impacted social structures:

1. *Rise of the middle class.* Industrialization led to the growth of the middle class as more people became entrepreneurs, professionals, and managers in the new industrial economy.

This created new social structures and power dynamics as the middle class emerged as a powerful force in society.

2. *Urbanization.* Industrialization also led to massive urbanization as people moved from rural areas to cities to work in factories. This led to the development of new social structures in urban areas, such as the rise of tenement housing, public transportation, and the emergence of new social classes.

3. *Division of labor.* Industrialization also led to the division of labor as specialized workers became necessary to operate complex machines and production processes. This led to the development of new social structures within workplaces, such as managers, supervisors, and workers.

4. *Social mobility.* Industrialization also created new opportunities for social mobility as people could move up the social ladder by acquiring new skills or starting their own businesses. This created new social structures based on merit and achievement rather than traditional social hierarchies.

5. *Family structures.* Industrialization also impacted family structures as people moved away from extended family networks and began to form smaller nuclear families. This had implications for child-rearing, education, and gender roles.

In summary, industrialization had a profound impact on social structures, leading to the rise of the middle class, massive urbanization, the division of labor, new opportunities for social mobility, and changes in family structures. These changes have had lasting implications for social organization and power dynamics in modern societies.

CHAPTER 3

The Biology of Connection

The neurological basis of human connection

HUMAN CONNECTION IS a complex and multifaceted phenomenon that has both psychological and neurological underpinnings. Neurologically speaking, human connection involves the activation of certain brain regions and neural networks that are responsible for social cognition and emotion regulation.

Research has shown that the neural basis of human connection involves several key brain regions and neural networks including the following:

1. *Mirror neuron system.* The mirror neuron system is a network of neurons that is activated when we observe others' actions and emotions. These neurons help us understand and empathize with others, and they play a critical role in social cognition and social learning.

2. *Prefrontal cortex.* The prefrontal cortex is the part of the brain that is responsible for executive function, decision-making, and social behavior. It plays a critical role in regulating emotions and social behavior and is involved in the formation of social bonds.

3. *Limbic system.* The limbic system is a group of brain structures that is involved in emotion regulation and motivation. It includes the amygdala, which is responsible for processing emotional stimuli, and the hippocampus, which is responsible for memory formation and recall.

4. *Oxytocin.* Oxytocin is a hormone that is released during social bonding and associated with feelings of trust, empathy, and generosity. It is believed to play a critical role in the formation of social bonds and often referred to as the *love hormone.*

5. *Dopamine.* Dopamine is a neurotransmitter that is associated with pleasure and reward. It is released during social interaction and believed to play a role in reinforcing social behavior.

In summary, the neurological basis of human connection involves the activation of several key brain regions and neural networks including the mirror neuron system, the prefrontal cortex, the limbic system, and the release of hormones and neurotransmitters, such as oxytocin and dopamine. Understanding the neurological basis of human connection can help us better understand the importance of social interaction and the impact of social isolation on our health and well-being.

The physiological effects of loneliness and isolation

Loneliness and social isolation can have significant physiological effects on the body, which can impact our health and well-being in a number of ways. Here are some of the physiological effects of loneliness and isolation:

1. *Increased inflammation.* Chronic loneliness and social isolation have been associated with increased levels of inflammation in the body. Inflammation is an immune response that can damage tissues and organs over time, increasing

the risk of chronic diseases, such as cardiovascular disease, diabetes, and cancer.

2. *Higher levels of stress hormones.* Loneliness and social isolation can also lead to higher levels of stress hormones, such as cortisol. Chronic stress can lead to a range of health problems including high blood pressure, heart disease, and depression.

3. *Weakened immune system.* Research has shown that loneliness and social isolation can weaken the immune system, making it more difficult for the body to fight off infections and illnesses.

4. *Sleep disturbances.* Loneliness and social isolation have been associated with sleep disturbances including difficulty falling asleep and staying asleep. Poor sleep can impact our physical and mental health, leading to fatigue, irritability, and reduced cognitive function.

5. *Altered gene expression.* Studies have found that loneliness and social isolation can alter the expression of genes involved in immune function, inflammation, and stress regulation, which can have negative health consequences.

In summary, loneliness and social isolation can have significant physiological effects on the body, impacting inflammation, stress hormones, the immune system, sleep, and gene expression. These effects can increase the risk of a range of health problems and highlight the importance of social connection for our health and well-being.

The impact of stress on physical health

Stress can have a significant impact on physical health, affecting various body systems and increasing the risk of a range of health problems. Here are some of the ways stress can impact physical health:

1. *Cardiovascular system.* Stress can lead to increased heart rate, blood pressure, and inflammation in the cardiovas-

cular system, which can increase the risk of heart disease, stroke, and other cardiovascular problems.

2. *Immune system.* Chronic stress can weaken the immune system, making it more difficult for the body to fight off infections and illnesses. This can increase the risk of a range of health problems including infections, autoimmune diseases, and cancer.

3. *Digestive system.* Stress can lead to a range of digestive problems including stomach ulcers, irritable bowel syndrome, and inflammatory bowel disease. Stress can also impact the gut microbiome, which can impact overall health and well-being.

4. *Respiratory system.* Stress can lead to increased inflammation and constriction in the airways, making it more difficult to breathe. This can worsen asthma and other respiratory conditions.

5. *Musculoskeletal system.* Stress can cause muscle tension, leading to headaches, neck and back pain, and other musculoskeletal problems. Chronic stress can also increase the risk of chronic pain conditions, such as fibromyalgia.

6. *Reproductive system.* Stress can impact the reproductive system, leading to menstrual irregularities, decreased fertility, and other reproductive problems.

In summary, stress can impact various body systems, increasing the risk of a range of health problems. Managing stress through techniques such as exercise, relaxation techniques, and social support can help mitigate these negative effects and promote overall health and well-being.

CHAPTER 4

The Psychological Effects of Isolation

The link between isolation and mental health

THERE IS A well-established link between social isolation and poor mental health. Studies have shown that social isolation and loneliness can increase the risk of a range of mental health problems, including depression, anxiety, and substance abuse. Here are some of the ways isolation can impact mental health:

1. *Depression.* Social isolation and loneliness can increase the risk of depression. Research has shown that people who are socially isolated are more likely to experience symptoms of depression and that social support can be an important factor in preventing and treating depression.
2. *Anxiety.* Social isolation can also increase the risk of anxiety. Social support and connection can provide a sense of security and help people cope with stress and anxiety.
3. *Substance abuse.* Social isolation has been linked to an increased risk of substance abuse. People who are socially

isolated may turn to drugs or alcohol as a way to cope with feelings of loneliness and depression.

4. *Cognitive decline.* Social isolation can also impact cognitive function, leading to a decline in memory and other cognitive abilities. This is especially true in older adults, who may be more vulnerable to the negative effects of social isolation.

5. *Suicidal ideation.* Social isolation has also been linked to an increased risk of suicidal ideation and behavior. People who are socially isolated may lack the social support and resources they need to cope with feelings of despair and hopelessness.

In summary, social isolation can have a significant impact on mental health, increasing the risk of depression, anxiety, substance abuse, cognitive decline, and suicidal ideation. It is important to address feelings of social isolation and loneliness through strategies—such as social support, connection, and therapy—to promote mental health and well-being.

The effects of loneliness on the brain

Loneliness can have significant effects on the brain, impacting both its structure and function. Here are some of the ways loneliness can impact the brain:

1. *Brain structure.* Studies have shown that chronic loneliness can lead to changes in the brain's structure, specifically in the gray matter of the prefrontal cortex, anterior cingulate cortex, insula, and amygdala. These areas of the brain are involved in social processing, emotion regulation, and stress response.

2. *Stress response.* Loneliness can activate the body's stress response, leading to increased levels of stress hormones, such as cortisol. Chronic activation of the stress response can have negative effects on the brain, leading to hippo-

campal atrophy and impaired memory and cognitive function.

3. *Emotion regulation.* Loneliness can impact the brain's ability to regulate emotions, leading to increased levels of negative emotions, such as sadness, anxiety, and anger. This can further exacerbate feelings of loneliness and social isolation.

4. *Reward processing.* Loneliness can impact the brain's reward processing system, leading to decreased activation in the ventral striatum and other areas of the brain involved in processing reward and pleasure. This can lead to a decrease in motivation and a decrease in the ability to experience pleasure.

5. *Cognitive function.* Loneliness can also impact cognitive function, specifically in the areas of attention, memory, and executive function. This can lead to impaired decision-making and decreased ability to perform tasks that require complex cognitive processing.

In summary, loneliness can have significant effects on the brain, impacting its structure and function in a number of ways. It is important to address feelings of loneliness and social isolation through strategies—such as social support, connection, and therapy—to promote brain health and overall well-being.

The role of relationships in psychological well-being

Relationships play a critical role in psychological well-being, and research has consistently shown that social connections are associated with better mental health outcomes. Here are some of the ways relationships can impact psychological well-being:

1. *Social support.* Relationships can provide social support, which can be an important buffer against stress and help people cope with difficult life events. Social support can come in many forms, such as emotional support, practical support, and informational support.

2. *Sense of belonging.* Relationships can provide a sense of belonging and connectedness, which is a fundamental human need. Feeling connected to others can help people feel valued, accepted, and part of a larger community.

3. *Self-esteem.* Relationships can impact self-esteem and self-worth, particularly when they involve positive feedback, encouragement, and validation. Feeling valued and appreciated by others can contribute to a sense of self-worth and confidence.

4. *Reduced loneliness and depression.* Relationships can reduce feelings of loneliness and depression, which can be particularly important for individuals who may be at risk for these conditions.

5. *Increased happiness.* Relationships can contribute to happiness and positive affect. Spending time with loved ones and engaging in activities with others can lead to positive emotions and an overall sense of well-being.

In summary, relationships can have a profound impact on psychological well-being. Social connections can provide support, a sense of belonging, self-esteem, and happiness while reducing feelings of loneliness and depression. It is important to prioritize and nurture relationships as a key component of maintaining good mental health.

CHAPTER 5

The Social Implications of Isolation

The impact of isolation on social skills

Isolation can have a significant impact on social skills, particularly for individuals who experience prolonged periods of social isolation. Here are some of the ways isolation can impact social skills:

1. *Reduced social interaction.* Isolation can limit opportunities for social interaction and lead to decreased social skills. Without opportunities to practice socializing and interacting with others, social skills can become rusty, leading to difficulties in communication, socializing, and building relationships.

2. *Social anxiety.* Isolation can contribute to social anxiety, which can impact social skills. Individuals who experience social anxiety may avoid social situations, leading to a lack of opportunities to practice social skills, and develop comfort in social settings.

3. *Decreased empathy.* Isolation can impact empathy, which is a critical component of social skills. When individuals

are isolated, they may have less exposure to others and less opportunity to develop empathy and understanding of others' perspectives.

4. *Impaired communication.* Isolation can impact communication skills, particularly in terms of verbal and nonverbal communication. Individuals who are isolated may have limited opportunities to practice communication and struggle with reading social cues or conveying their own thoughts and feelings.

5. *Decreased confidence.* Isolation can impact confidence, which is an important component of social skills. When individuals are isolated, they may have fewer opportunities to receive positive feedback and validation, which can impact self-esteem and confidence in social situations.

The effects of loneliness on behavior

Loneliness can have a significant impact on behavior, and research has shown that loneliness is associated with a range of negative behavioral outcomes. Here are some of the ways loneliness can impact behavior:

1. *Increased social withdrawal.* Loneliness can lead to increased social withdrawal and avoidance of social situations. Individuals who feel lonely may be less likely to initiate social interactions or seek out opportunities for social connection.

2. *Increased substance use.* Loneliness can contribute to increased substance use, including alcohol and drug use. Individuals who feel lonely may turn to substances as a way of coping with their feelings of isolation and disconnection.

3. *Reduced physical activity.* Loneliness can contribute to reduced physical activity as individuals may be less motivated to engage in physical activities when they feel disconnected and unmotivated.

4. *Increased risk-taking behavior*. Loneliness can lead to increased risk-taking behavior as individuals may be less concerned with the consequences of their actions when they feel isolated and disconnected.

5. *Aggression and hostility*. Loneliness can contribute to feelings of frustration and irritability, which can lead to increased aggression and hostility.

In summary, loneliness can impact behavior in a number of ways, leading to increased social withdrawal, substance use, reduced physical activity, increased risk-taking behavior, and aggression and hostility. It is important to address feelings of loneliness and seek out opportunities for social connection as a way of mitigating these negative behavioral outcomes.

The connection between isolation and aggression

Isolation can be connected to increased aggression and hostility in individuals, and research has shown that there is a relationship between social isolation and aggressive behavior. Here are some ways isolation can impact aggression:

1. *Increased feelings of frustration and irritability*. When individuals are isolated, they may experience increased feelings of frustration and irritability, which can contribute to aggressive behavior.

2. *Decreased social support*. Without a support system to turn to, individuals may feel more vulnerable, which can lead to a defensive response and aggressive behavior.

3. *Reduced empathy*. Isolation can impact empathy, which is a critical component of understanding and empathizing with others. Without exposure to social situations and opportunities to practice empathy, individuals may be more likely to act aggressively towards others.

4. *Negative self-talk*. Isolation can contribute to negative self-talk, which can impact mood and behavior. Individuals

who are isolated may engage in negative self-talk, which can lead to feelings of anger and aggression toward others.

5. *Social learning.* Social isolation can lead to an increased focus on media and other forms of communication that may promote aggressive behavior or attitudes.

In summary, social isolation can lead to increased aggression and hostility in individuals. By understanding the link between isolation and aggression, individuals can take steps to address feelings of isolation and seek out opportunities for social connection as a way of mitigating these negative outcomes.

CHAPTER 6

The Benefits of Relationships

The positive effects of social support

SOCIAL SUPPORT CAN have many positive effects on individuals, including:

1. *Reduced stress.* Social support can help individuals manage stress, reducing the negative impact that stress can have on physical and mental health.
2. *Improved mood.* Social support can boost mood and reduce feelings of anxiety and depression.
3. *Increased self-esteem.* Social support can provide a sense of validation and positive feedback, which can boost self-esteem and confidence.
4. *Improved physical health.* Social support has been linked to improved physical health outcomes, such as a lower risk of chronic diseases, like heart disease and diabetes.
5. *Improved coping skills.* Social support can help individuals develop and improve coping skills, which can help them to manage challenging situations and overcome adversity.
6. *Increased sense of belonging.* Social support can help individuals feel a sense of belonging and connection, which is important for overall well-being.

7. *Increased motivation.* Social support can help individuals set and achieve goals, providing motivation and account-ability.

In summary, social support can have many positive effects on individuals, including reduced stress, improved mood, increased self-esteem, improved physical health, improved coping skills, increased sense of belonging, and increased motivation. It is import-ant for individuals to seek out and cultivate social support networks as a way of promoting overall well-being.

The role of relationships in personal growth

Relationships can play a significant role in personal growth and development. Here are some ways relationships can impact personal growth:

1. *Providing feedback.* Relationships can provide individuals with feedback about their strengths and areas for improve-ment, which can help facilitate personal growth.
2. *Encouraging self-reflection.* Relationships can encourage individuals to engage in self-reflection and introspection, which is an important component of personal growth.
3. *Providing support.* Relationships can provide emotional and practical support, which can help individuals overcome challenges and reach their goals.
4. *Challenging beliefs and assumptions.* Relationships can chal-lenge individuals' beliefs and assumptions, which can help them broaden their perspective and expand their world-view.
5. *Facilitating learning and development.* Relationships can provide opportunities for learning and development as individuals can learn from others' experiences and perspec-tives.
6. *Providing accountability.* Relationships can provide accountability as individuals may be more motivated to

follow through on goals and commitments when they know that others are counting on them.

7. *Fostering a sense of purpose.* Relationships can foster a sense of purpose and meaning, which can contribute to personal growth and well-being.

In summary, relationships can play a critical role in personal growth, providing feedback, encouraging self-reflection, providing support, challenging beliefs and assumptions, facilitating learning and development, providing accountability, and fostering a sense of purpose. It is important for individuals to cultivate positive and supportive relationships as a way of promoting personal growth and well-being.

The importance of emotional connections

Emotional connections are important for many reasons including the following:

1. *Improved mental health.* Emotional connections can promote positive mental health by providing individuals with a sense of support, validation, and belonging.
2. *Enhanced well-being.* Emotional connections can increase feelings of happiness, satisfaction, and fulfillment in life.
3. *Greater resilience.* Emotional connections can help individuals cope with adversity and bounce back from difficult situations.
4. *Improved physical health.* Emotional connections have been linked to improved physical health outcomes, such as lower blood pressure and a reduced risk of chronic diseases.
5. *Better communication skills.* Emotional connections can help individuals develop and improve their communication skills, which can benefit their personal and professional relationships.
6. *Increased empathy and compassion.* Emotional connections can help individuals develop greater empathy and compas-

sion for others, which can enhance relationships and promote social cohesion.

7. *Increased self-awareness.* Emotional connections can promote self-awareness as individuals may gain insights into their own emotions and behaviors through their interactions with others.

In summary, emotional connections are important for promoting positive mental and physical health, enhancing well-being, building resilience, improving communication skills, increasing empathy and compassion, and promoting self-awareness. It is important for individuals to cultivate and maintain emotional connections with others as a way of promoting overall well-being.

CHAPTER 7

Romantic Relationships

The impact of isolation on romantic relationships

Isolation can have a significant impact on romantic relationships in a number of ways. Here are some examples:

1. *Communication breakdown.* Isolation can lead to communication breakdown between partners. When individuals are physically or emotionally distant from their partner, it can be difficult to communicate effectively or maintain the emotional connection that is essential to a healthy relationship.
2. *Increased conflict.* Isolation can lead to increased conflict between partners. When individuals feel disconnected or isolated, they may become more defensive, critical, or distant, which can lead to arguments and misunderstandings.
3. *Reduced intimacy.* Isolation can lead to a reduction in intimacy between partners. When individuals feel disconnected from their partner, they may be less likely to engage in physical or emotional intimacy, which can further strain the relationship.
4. *Decreased emotional support.* Isolation can lead to a decrease in emotional support within the relationship. When indi-

viduals are isolated, they may not have the emotional support that they need from their partner, which can lead to feelings of loneliness or even depression.

5. *Decreased trust.* Isolation can lead to a decrease in trust between partners. When both individuals feel disconnected or isolated from their partner, they may be more likely to feel suspicious or mistrustful of their partner's intentions or actions.

6. *Increased infidelity.* Isolation can increase the likelihood of infidelity within the relationship. When individuals feel disconnected or isolated from their partner, they may be more likely to seek emotional or physical connection elsewhere.

In summary, isolation can have a significant impact on romantic relationships, leading to communication breakdown, increased conflict, reduced intimacy, decreased emotional support, decreased trust, and increased infidelity. It is important for couples to prioritize their relationship and work to maintain emotional connection, even during times of stress or isolation. This can involve open and honest communication, intentional efforts to maintain intimacy, and a focus on building trust and emotional support within the relationship.

The benefits of healthy relationships

Healthy relationships offer a wide range of benefits to individuals, including the following:

1. *Improved mental health.* Healthy relationships can provide individuals with a sense of support, validation, and belonging, which can promote positive mental health outcomes.

2. *Increased happiness and life satisfaction.* Healthy relationships can increase feelings of happiness, satisfaction, and fulfillment in life.

3. *Greater resilience.* Healthy relationships can help individuals cope with adversity and bounce back from difficult situations.
4. *Improved physical health.* Healthy relationships have been linked to improved physical health outcomes, such as lower blood pressure and a reduced risk of chronic diseases.
5. *Better communication skills.* Healthy relationships can help individuals develop and improve their communication skills, which can benefit their personal and professional relationships.
6. *Increased empathy and compassion.* Healthy relationships can help individuals develop greater empathy and compassion for others, which can enhance relationships and promote social cohesion.
7. *Increased self-awareness.* Healthy relationships can promote self-awareness as individuals may gain insights into their own emotions and behaviors through their interactions with others.
8. *Improved personal growth.* Healthy relationships can provide individuals with opportunities for personal growth and self-improvement through feedback, guidance, and support from their partner.

In summary, healthy relationships can promote positive mental and physical health outcomes, enhance well-being, build resilience, improve communication skills, increase empathy and compassion, promote self-awareness, and foster personal growth. It is important for individuals to cultivate and maintain healthy relationships in their personal and professional lives as a way of promoting overall well-being.

The importance of communication and empathy

Communication and empathy are two essential components of healthy relationships; and they play a crucial role in promoting understanding, trust, and connection between individuals.

Communication involves the exchange of thoughts, feelings, and ideas between individuals, and it is necessary for building and maintaining healthy relationships. Effective communication requires active listening, the ability to express oneself clearly and honestly, and a willingness to compromise and find common ground.

Empathy, on the other hand, involves the ability to understand and share the feelings of others. Empathy is essential for building strong emotional connections and promoting mutual understanding and respect. By practicing empathy, individuals can better understand the perspectives and experiences of others, which can lead to more harmonious relationships and improved problem-solving.

Effective communication and empathy work together to promote healthy relationships. When individuals communicate effectively, they are better able to express their needs and feelings and understand the needs and feelings of their partner. Empathy helps individuals connect with their partner on a deeper emotional level, leading to greater trust, respect, and intimacy.

In addition to promoting healthy relationships, communication and empathy can have positive impacts on personal and professional relationships as well as mental and physical health. Individuals who communicate effectively and practice empathy may be better equipped to handle conflicts, reduce stress, and improve overall well-being.

In summary, communication and empathy are essential components of healthy relationships. By practicing effective communication and empathy, individuals can build stronger emotional connections, promote understanding and respect, and improve their overall well-being.

CHAPTER 8

Friendship

The importance of friendship in adult life

FRIENDSHIP IS AN important aspect of adult life, and it can provide individuals with numerous benefits that can enhance their overall well-being. Some of the key reasons that friendship is important in adult life include the following:

1. *Social support.* Friends provide social support during both good times and bad. They can offer encouragement, empathy, and advice and help individuals feel less alone and more connected.
2. *Stress relief.* Spending time with friends can be an effective way to reduce stress and promote relaxation. Engaging in fun activities with friends can also provide a welcome break from the daily grind of work and other responsibilities.
3. *Increased happiness.* Having close friendships can contribute to increased feelings of happiness and life satisfaction. Friendships can provide a sense of belonging and connectedness and contribute to a more positive outlook on life.
4. *Improved mental health.* Friendships have been linked to improved mental health outcomes, such as lower levels of depression and anxiety. Having a strong social support net-

work can help individuals cope with difficult life events and challenges.

5. *Healthier behaviors.* Friends can have a positive influence on one another's behaviors, encouraging healthy habits (such as exercise or healthy eating) and avoiding negative behaviors (such as smoking or excessive drinking).

6. *Opportunities for personal growth.* Friendships can offer opportunities for personal growth and learning. Friends can provide feedback, support, and guidance and challenge one another to try new things and take on new challenges.

In summary, friendship is an important aspect of adult life that can provide numerous benefits. By fostering close friendships, individuals can enjoy social support, stress relief, increased happiness, improved mental health, healthier behaviors, and opportunities for personal growth. It is important for individuals to prioritize friendship in their lives and make time for meaningful connections with others.

The impact of social networks on health

Social networks can have both positive and negative impacts on health, depending on how they are used. Here are some ways social networks can affect health:

1. Positive impacts

    a. *Social support.* Social networks can provide emotional support and a sense of community, which can have a positive impact on mental health. People can connect with others who share similar experiences and offer support, and they can receive encouragement during difficult times.

    b. *Health information.* Social networks can be a valuable source of health information, allowing people to learn about new treatments, medical breakthroughs, and ways to stay healthy.

c. *Awareness*. Social networks can increase awareness about important health issues, such as the importance of exercise, healthy eating, and regular checkups.

2. Negative impacts

   a. *Cyberbullying*. Social networks can facilitate cyberbullying, which can have a negative impact on mental health, causing anxiety, depression, and even suicidal thoughts.
   b. *Addiction*. Social networks can be addictive, leading to excessive use and the neglect of other important activities, such as exercise and social interaction in person.
   c. *Comparing oneself to others*. Social networks can create feelings of inadequacy and low self-esteem as people often compare themselves to others who seem to have a better life or appearance.

Overall, social networks can have a significant impact on health, but it is important to use them mindfully—in a way that maximizes the positive aspects and minimizes the negative ones.

The value of shared experiences and memories

Shared experiences and memories are valuable because they help build and strengthen relationships among individuals. Here are some reasons that shared experiences and memories are important:

1. *Connection*. Shared experiences and memories can create a sense of connection among people. By going through an experience together, individuals can feel a sense of solidarity and shared purpose.
2. *Understanding*. Shared experiences and memories can help individuals understand one another better. When peo-

ple share their experiences, they can gain insight into one another's perspectives and values, which can lead to greater empathy and understanding.

3. *Nostalgia.* Shared memories can create a sense of nostalgia that brings people together. By reminiscing about past experiences, people can feel a sense of shared history and shared identity, which can be comforting and enjoyable.

4. *Bonding.* Shared experiences and memories can create strong bonds among people. When people share a meaningful experience, they can feel a sense of camaraderie and loyalty that can last a lifetime.

5. *Support.* Shared experiences and memories can provide support during difficult times. When people have gone through a challenging experience together, they can offer one another emotional support and understanding.

Overall, shared experiences and memories are important because they help create meaningful connections among people, foster empathy and understanding, and provide a source of comfort and support during challenging times.

CHAPTER 9

Parenting and Family Relationships

The role of family relationships in child development

FAMILY RELATIONSHIPS PLAY a crucial role in child development. Here are some ways family relationships can impact a child's development:

1. *Emotional development.* The emotional support provided by family members is critical to a child's emotional development. Children need to feel loved, safe, and secure to develop healthy emotional and social skills.

2. *Cognitive development.* Family interactions and conversations can impact a child's cognitive development. Children who engage in frequent conversations with their family members tend to have better language and communication skills.

3. *Social development.* Family relationships are an important aspect of a child's social development. Children who have positive relationships with their family members are more

likely to develop healthy social skills, such as sharing, taking turns, and cooperation.

4. *Self-esteem.* Family relationships can also impact a child's self-esteem. Children who feel loved, valued, and supported by their family members tend to have higher self-esteem and greater confidence in themselves.

5. *Behavior.* The quality of family relationships can also impact a child's behavior. Children who have stable and supportive family relationships are less likely to engage in risky behaviors or have emotional and behavioral problems.

Overall, family relationships play a crucial role in a child's development. A supportive and loving family can provide children with a strong foundation for healthy emotional, cognitive, social, and behavioral development.

The importance of supportive parenting

Supportive parenting is critical for a child's healthy development. Here are some reasons that supportive parenting is important:

1. *Emotional well-being.* Supportive parenting helps foster emotional well-being in children. Children who have supportive parents tend to have lower rates of depression, anxiety, and other emotional problems.

2. *Self-esteem.* Supportive parenting helps build children's self-esteem. Children who feel loved, valued, and supported by their parents tend to have higher self-esteem and a greater sense of self-worth.

3. *Cognitive development.* Supportive parenting helps promote cognitive development. Children who receive positive feedback and encouragement from their parents tend to have better cognitive skills, such as memory, attention, and problem-solving.

4. *Behavior.* Supportive parenting helps encourage positive behavior in children. Children who have supportive par-

ents are more likely to engage in prosocial behavior, such as sharing and helping others.

5. *Resilience.* Supportive parenting helps to foster resilience in children. Children who have supportive parents are better able to cope with stress and adversity and more likely to have a positive outlook on life.

Overall, supportive parenting is critical for a child's healthy development. It helps promote emotional well-being, self-esteem, cognitive development, positive behavior, and resilience. Parents who provide a supportive and loving environment for their children are helping them build a strong foundation for a happy and healthy life.

The impact of isolation on children

Isolation can have a negative impact on children's development and well-being. Here are some ways isolation can affect children:

1. *Social skills.* Isolation can limit opportunities for children to interact with peers and develop social skills. Children who are isolated may struggle to make friends, communicate effectively, and develop healthy relationships with others.
2. *Emotional well-being.* Isolation can also have a negative impact on children's emotional well-being. Children who are isolated may feel lonely, sad, and anxious. They may also be at a higher risk of developing depression and other emotional problems.
3. *Cognitive development.* Isolation can limit children's opportunities to learn and develop cognitive skills. Children who are isolated may have fewer opportunities to engage in stimulating activities, such as play, exploration, and problem-solving.
4. *Physical health.* Isolation can also have a negative impact on children's physical health. Children who are isolated may be less physically active and have poorer health outcomes.

5. *Risk of abuse.* Isolated children may be at a higher risk of abuse as they may have fewer opportunities to interact with trusted adults who could identify and report abuse.

Overall, isolation can have a negative impact on children's development and well-being. It can limit opportunities for social interaction and cognitive development, increase the risk of emotional and physical problems, and put children at a higher risk of abuse. It is important to ensure that children have opportunities to interact with peers and trusted adults as well as identify and address any concerns related to isolation.

CHAPTER 10

The Importance of Communities

The benefits of community involvement

COMMUNITY INVOLVEMENT CAN bring a variety of benefits to both individuals and the community as a whole. Here are some benefits of community involvement:

1. *Social connections.* Community involvement can help individuals build social connections and develop a sense of belonging. This can help combat loneliness and isolation, which can have negative effects on mental health.
2. *Skill development.* Community involvement can provide individuals with opportunities to learn new skills and gain experience in areas that interest them. This can help build self-confidence and increase employability.
3. *Positive impact.* Community involvement allows individuals to make a positive impact on their community. This can help increase feelings of purpose and satisfaction in life and contribute to a sense of civic responsibility.
4. *Networking.* Community involvement can provide opportunities for individuals to meet and connect with people who share similar interests and goals. This can help build

professional and personal networks that can be useful in the future.

5. *Health benefits.* Community involvement can have positive effects on physical health, such as reducing the risk of chronic diseases and improving overall well-being. It can also provide opportunities for physical activity and healthy social interactions.

Overall, community involvement can bring a range of benefits to both individuals and the community as a whole. It can help build social connections, provide opportunities for skill development, create a positive impact, foster networking, and promote physical and mental health.

The impact of communities on individual well-being

Communities can have a significant impact on individual well-being. Here are some ways communities can impact well-being:

1. *Social connections.* Communities provide individuals with opportunities to develop social connections and a sense of belonging. This can help combat feelings of loneliness and isolation, which can have negative effects on mental health.
2. *Emotional support.* Communities can provide emotional support to individuals during difficult times, such as through loss or illness. This support can help individuals cope with stress and build resilience.
3. *Sense of purpose.* Communities can provide individuals with a sense of purpose and meaning in life. This can help increase feelings of satisfaction and fulfillment and reduce the risk of depression and other emotional problems.
4. *Access to resources.* Communities can provide individuals with access to resources, such as health care, education, and job opportunities. This can improve overall well-being and increase opportunities for personal growth and development.

5. *Positive role models.* Communities can provide individuals with positive role models and examples to follow. This can help build self-esteem and confidence and encourage positive behaviors.

Overall, communities can have a significant impact on individual well-being. They can provide social connections, emotional support, a sense of purpose, access to resources, and positive role models. By fostering a strong sense of community, individuals can build a foundation for a happy and healthy life.

The role of communities in creating social change

Communities play a vital role in creating social change. Here are some ways communities can influence and promote social change:

1. *Collective action.* Communities can organize collective action to bring about change. By working together, community members can pool their resources and knowledge to address social issues and create positive change.
2. *Advocacy.* Communities can advocate for change by raising awareness and engaging in public education. By spreading the word and increasing understanding of an issue, community members can build support for social change.
3. *Grassroots organizing.* Community can engage in grassroots organizing, which involves mobilizing community members at the local level to work toward social change. By building strong networks and coalitions, community members can leverage their collective power to bring about change.
4. *Political action.* Communities can engage in political action by supporting policies and candidates that align with their values and promote social change. By organizing and engaging in political campaigns, community members can have a significant impact on policy and legislation.

5. *Social norms.* Communities can influence social norms by promoting values and beliefs that support social change. By creating a culture of support for social change, community members can encourage others to join their cause and create a positive ripple effect.

Overall, communities play a crucial role in creating social change. By organizing collective action, advocating for change, engaging in grassroots organizing, engaging in political action, and influencing social norms, community members can have a significant impact on the world around them.

CHAPTER 11

Overcoming Isolation and Loneliness

The importance of seeking social connections

Seeking social connections is important for overall well-being and has many benefits. Here are some reasons that seeking social connections is important:

1. *Reduced loneliness.* Social connections provide a sense of belonging and reduce feelings of loneliness. Loneliness has been linked to various negative health outcomes, such as depression and anxiety.

2. *Improved mental health.* Social connections can improve mental health by providing emotional support and reducing stress. Having someone to talk to and share experiences with can help individuals cope with difficult situations and build resilience.

3. *Increased happiness.* Social connections can increase happiness by providing opportunities for fun, laughter, and positive experiences. Building connections with others can

create positive memories and experiences that can enhance well-being.

4. *Improved physical health.* Social connections have been linked to improved physical health outcomes, such as lower rates of chronic disease and better immune function. This may be due to the positive effect of social connections on stress levels and other health behaviors.

5. *Networking.* Social connections provide opportunities for networking and career advancement. Building connections with others can create professional opportunities and enhance employability.

Overall, seeking social connections is important for overall well-being. It can reduce loneliness, improve mental and physical health, increase happiness, and provide opportunities for networking and career advancement. By investing in social connections, individuals can build a foundation for a happy and fulfilling life.

The role of therapy and counseling

Therapy and counseling can play an important role in promoting mental health and well-being. Here are some ways therapy and counseling can be beneficial:

1. *Addressing mental health concerns.* Therapy and counseling can be effective in treating mental health concerns, such as depression, anxiety, post-traumatic stress disorder, and addiction. These conditions can negatively impact an individual's well-being, and therapy can provide a supportive and safe environment to address these issues.

2. *Providing coping strategies.* Therapy and counseling can provide individuals with coping strategies to manage stress, improve communication, and handle difficult situations. By learning new coping skills, individuals can build resilience and improve their overall well-being.

3. *Supporting personal growth.* Therapy and counseling can be used to support personal growth and development. Through therapy, individuals can explore their own values, beliefs, and behaviors and gain insight into themselves. This can lead to increased self-awareness and self-acceptance.
4. *Improving relationships.* Therapy and counseling can help individuals to improve their relationships with others. By learning better communication and conflict resolution skills, individuals can improve their relationships with partners, family members, and coworkers.
5. Providing a safe and supportive environment: Therapy and counseling provide a safe and confidential environment where individuals can share their thoughts and feelings. This can be particularly beneficial for those who feel isolated or unsupported in their daily lives.

Overall, therapy and counseling can play an important role in promoting mental health and well-being. By addressing mental health concerns, providing coping strategies, supporting personal growth, improving relationships, and providing a safe and supportive environment, therapy and counseling can help individuals live happier and more fulfilling lives.

The benefits of group therapy and support groups

Group therapy and support groups can be beneficial for individuals seeking to improve their mental health and overall well-being. Here are some benefits of group therapy and support groups:

1. *Increased social support.* Group therapy and support groups provide individuals with a supportive community of peers who are going through similar experiences. This can reduce feelings of isolation and provide a sense of belonging.
2. *Learning from others.* Group therapy and support groups provide opportunities for individuals to learn from the

experiences of others. Hearing others' stories can provide insight, perspective, and a sense of empathy and understanding.

3. *Improved communication and social skills.* Group therapy and support groups provide a safe and supportive environment to practice communication and social skills. Through group interaction and feedback, individuals can improve their social skills and learn to better express themselves.

4. *Reduced sense of shame.* Group therapy and support groups can reduce feelings of shame and stigma associated with mental health concerns. By seeing others who are going through similar experiences, individuals can feel more accepting of their own struggles.

5. *Lower costs.* Group therapy and support groups can be a more cost-effective option than individual therapy, making it more accessible to those with limited resources.

Overall, group therapy and support groups can be beneficial for individuals seeking to improve their mental health and overall well-being. By providing increased social support, opportunities to learn from others, improved communication and social skills, reduced sense of shame, and lower costs, group therapy and support groups can help individuals build a sense of community and work toward a healthier, more fulfilling life.

CHAPTER 12

Conclusion

The importance of social connections for men and women

SOCIAL CONNECTIONS ARE important for both men and women and can have a positive impact on mental and physical health, well-being, and quality of life. However, men and women may experience social connections differently due to societal norms, cultural expectations, and individual differences. Here are some ways social connections may be important for men and women:

1. *Women.* Research suggests that women may place a greater emphasis on relationships and social connections than men. Women are more likely to seek out emotional support and engage in social interactions that involve talking and sharing personal experiences. Women may also benefit more from social connections in terms of reduced stress and improved mental health outcomes.

2. *Men.* Men may be more likely to form social connections around shared activities, such as sports or hobbies. Men may also benefit from social connections in terms of improved physical health outcomes, such as lower rates of heart disease and mortality. However, men may be less likely to seek out emotional support or express their feel-

ings openly, which can make it more difficult to form close relationships.

Overall, social connections are important for both men and women and can have a positive impact on well-being and quality of life. While men and women may experience social connections differently, it is important for both to prioritize building and maintaining social connections that are supportive, fulfilling, and meaningful.

The benefits of healthy relationships

Healthy relationships can have a positive impact on physical and mental health, overall well-being, and quality of life. Here are some benefits of healthy relationships:

1. *Improved mental health.* Healthy relationships can provide emotional support, reduce stress, and increase feelings of happiness and contentment. Positive relationships can also promote a sense of belonging, purpose, and meaning in life.
2. *Reduced risk of health problems.* Healthy relationships can reduce the risk of health problems, such as depression, anxiety, and cardiovascular disease. Individuals in healthy relationships may also have better immune-system functioning and lower rates of chronic illnesses.
3. *Increased longevity.* Research suggests that individuals in healthy relationships may live longer than those who are isolated or in unhealthy relationships. Social support and emotional connection can provide a sense of purpose and meaning, which can contribute to a longer and healthier life.
4. *Improved communication and conflict-resolution skills.* Healthy relationships provide opportunities to practice communication and conflict-resolution skills, which can be useful in other areas of life, such as work or other relationships.

5. *Greater personal growth.* Healthy relationships can provide opportunities for personal growth and development. Partners or close friends can provide honest feedback, challenge negative patterns, and encourage self-reflection and self-improvement.

Overall, healthy relationships can have a positive impact on physical and mental health, overall well-being, and quality of life. By providing emotional support, reducing stress, promoting a sense of belonging, reducing the risk of health problems, increasing longevity, improving communication and conflict-resolution skills, and promoting personal growth, healthy relationships can contribute to a happier, healthier, and more fulfilling life.

The power of communities in creating a better world

Communities can be powerful forces for creating positive change in the world. Here are some ways communities can create a better world:

1. *Collective action.* When people come together for a common cause or issue, they can use their collective power to effect change. Through organizing, protesting, and advocating for change, communities can raise awareness and influence policy to improve the lives of individuals and communities.
2. *Mutual support.* Communities can provide emotional and practical support to individuals in need. This can include offering financial assistance, providing meals, or offering a helping hand to those going through difficult times.
3. *Sharing resources.* Communities can share resources and knowledge to help improve the lives of all members. This can include sharing information about health and wellness, providing access to community gardens or resources for those in need, or offering education and training programs.

4. *Fostering diversity and inclusivity.* By creating spaces that are welcoming and inclusive, communities can help break down barriers and promote diversity and acceptance. By valuing and embracing differences, communities can work toward creating a more equitable and just world for all.

5. *Inspiring positive change.* Communities can inspire individuals to make positive changes in their own lives and communities. By modeling positive behaviors, values, and attitudes, communities can encourage others to make positive changes in their own lives and contribute to a better world.

Overall, communities can be powerful forces for creating positive change in the world. By coming together for common causes, providing mutual support, sharing resources, fostering diversity and inclusivity, and inspiring positive change, communities can work toward creating a more just, equitable, and compassionate world for all.

Social Tweet

I AM a True Believer that it's NOT Good for Man to be Alone (includes women) and therefore authoring a book titled "The ABC's of Why It is NOT GOOD for Man to Be Alone" and sharing excerpts as a modern day series here. I hope you enjoy! (@LouisDace)

Louis Dace is a highly accomplished and successful American entrepreneur making his mark as an influential leader in the world of technology. Blessed with determination and a relentless drive to succeed, Louis has built a remarkable career in the rapidly growing industries of artificial intelligence, cloud computing, computer vision, CCTV, Internet of Things, and on-demand intelligent video analytics.

As the founder and CEO of Dace IT LLC, operating under the brand name Sense Traffic Pulse, Louis has established himself as a true visionary in the field. His dedication to innovation and excellence has led to fruitful partnerships with some of the world's most renowned technology companies, including Apple, Amazon, Axis Communications, Google, IBM, Intel, and Microsoft.

Throughout his illustrious career, Louis Dace has consistently demonstrated his ability to stay ahead of the curve, developing cutting-edge solutions to complex problems and delivering them to clients worldwide. As a result, he has earned a reputation as a twenty-first-century technology business tycoon, leaving an indelible mark on the industry.

In his unwavering pursuit of success, Louis serves as an inspiration to aspiring entrepreneurs and established professionals alike, proving that with hard work and persistence, anyone can achieve greatness. His story serves as a testament to the power of ambition and the limitless potential of human ingenuity.

www.ingramcontent.com/pod-product-compliance
Lightning Source LLC
Chambersburg PA
CBHW021811150726
47989CB00004B/1880